FOODS HIGHLY RICH IN VITAMIN D AND THEIR DOSAGE

Knowing the holistic function of vitamin D

BY

Dr DOUGLAS JASON

TABLE OF CONTENT

ABOUT THE AUTHOR

INTRODUCTION

TABLE OF CONTENTS

FOODS HIGHLY RICH IN VITAMIN D AND THEIR DOSAGE

Knowing the holistic function of vitamin D

INTRODUCTION

CHAPTER 1
Orange juice

CHAPTER 2
: Rainbow Trout

CHAPTER 3
Salmon

CHAPTER 4
Portobello mushrooms

CHAPTER 5
Yogurt

CHAPTER 6
Tuna

CHAPTER 7
Milk.

CHAPTER 8

Nondairy Milks

CHAPTER 9
Risk Factors for Low Vitamin D

CONCLUSIONS

Dr. Douglas Jason is a certified dietician who has a strong passion for wellness and a big eagerness to help people all over the world. He uses healthy food, herbs, spices, and other useful tools to help mankind realize its overall goal of optimum health.

INTRODUCTION

Why Vitamin D Is Important
Your immune system, blood cells, and bones are crucial for your body's fight against pathogens. Most of your vitamin D comes from exposure to sunshine on your skin. It should work with just a few minutes per day on your hands and face. However, food can also provide it. You might not get enough vitamin D if you're elderly, unwell, or housebound. If you believe that your levels are low, consult your doctor. What Quantity Do You Need?

The average adult requires 15 micrograms (mcg) each day. For babies, this decreases to 10 mcg, and for adults 71 and older, it increases to 20 mcg. You can encounter vitamin D amounts given in international units on labels (IU). 40 international units are equal to one microgram.

CHAPTER 1

Orange juice

In this instance, purchasing it from a retailer is preferable to manually pressing the product. This is because vitamin D is added to the juice at the factory and not taken directly from the oranges themselves. On the label, look for the phrase "enriched with vitamin D." Each cup yields roughly 2.5 mcg.

Don't drink too much orange juice, but do enjoy a glass. It is loaded with calories and sweets in addition to nutrients.

CHAPTER 2

: Rainbow Trout

Try grilling some rainbow trout if you're looking for a balanced main dish with plenty of vitamin D. In a 3-ounce serving, there are 16 mcg. For a great lunch, combine some butter, lemon, and herbs.

CHAPTER 3

Salmon

Depending on the mixture, a 3-ounce portion of salmon can provide you with 10 to 18 mcg of vitamin D. 10 mcg of wild coho salmon is at the low end, whereas 18 mcg of canned sockeye salmon is at the high end. The vitamin D range of other fatty fish like mackerel, herring, and sardines is also rather high.

Try baking salmon from a can with fish cakes for a quick supper.

CHAPTER 4

Portobello mushrooms

When you consume 3 ounces of portabella mushrooms, you can obtain 8 mg of vitamin D. However, you might take them outside so they can briefly view the sun. This is because sunlight's UV rays increase the amount of vitamin D in many mushrooms, especially portabellas.

Cook portabella mushrooms on the grill as an alternative to a meat meal by brushing them with olive oil.

CHAPTER 5

Yogurt

Vitamin D is frequently included in yogurt production. Typically, an 8-ounce serving contains 3 mcg. Choose plain, low-fat yogurt to consume fewer calories, sugar, and fat.

Cover fresh berries with plain, low-fat yogurt and crumbled almonds for a nutritious snack.

CHAPTER 6

Tuna

When compared to other foods, the inexpensive light tuna in a can carries a respectable amount of vitamin D. A 3-ounce serving provides 6 mcg.

To make a sandwich healthy, consider replacing the mayo with a concoction of Dijon mustard, olive oil, and lemon juice.

CHAPTER 7

Milk.

No matter if it is full, chocolate, or low-fat, the manufacturer probably included 3 mcg of vitamin D in each cup. Which kind should you choose, then, if you have a choice? (Hint: The chocolate isn't to blame.)

That's right, low-fat is the way to go. Try some the next morning with whole-grain, low-sugar cereal that has been vitamin D enriched frequently.

CHAPTER 8

Nondairy Milks

Producers often add 2.5 to 3 mcg of vitamin D per cup to goods manufactured from soy, almonds, or rice. Check the label carefully because these beverages can occasionally have a lot of calories, sugar, and fat as well.

A cup of almond milk will give your post-workout smoothie some nondairy smoothness.

CHAPTER 9

Risk Factors for Low Vitamin D

You're more likely to have low vitamin D levels if several factors exist:

Age: As you get older, your skin and kidneys don't function as well.
Darker skin: It is less effective at converting sunlight.
Your levels may be restricted by digestive issues such as Crohn's disease, celiac disease, and issues with fat digestion.

<u>Obesity:</u> Fat traps some vitamin D and prevents blood levels from rising.

CONCLUSIONS

Are You Vitamin D Deficient? Your blood can be tested by a doctor to determine your vitamin D levels. If you don't go outside or exhibit symptoms of low vitamin D, such as osteoporosis or soreness in your muscles or bones, you should think about getting one. Anything greater than 20 nanograms per milliliter (ng/mL) is considered typical for adults. Less than 12 may indicate a health issue.

Supplements may be beneficial, but see your doctor first and avoid going overboard. A hazardous level of vitamin D would be one over 100 ng/mL.